Mourad Raiah

Can myocardial infarction be predicted in cardiac emergencies?

Mourad Raiah

Can myocardial infarction be predicted in cardiac emergencies?

ScienciaScripts

Imprint

Any brand names and product names mentioned in this book are subject to trademark, brand or patent protection and are trademarks or registered trademarks of their respective holders. The use of brand names, product names, common names, trade names, product descriptions etc. even without a particular marking in this work is in no way to be construed to mean that such names may be regarded as unrestricted in respect of trademark and brand protection legislation and could thus be used by anyone.

Cover image: www.ingimage.com

This book is a translation from the original published under ISBN 978-620-6-71158-2.

Publisher:
Sciencia Scripts
is a trademark of
Dodo Books Indian Ocean Ltd. and OmniScriptum S.R.L publishing group

120 High Road, East Finchley, London, N2 9ED, United Kingdom
Str. Armeneasca 28/1, office 1, Chisinau MD-2012, Republic of Moldova, Europe
Printed at: see last page
ISBN: 978-620-7-63674-7

1. Introduction

Myocardial infarction (MI) is an absolute cardiological emergency, the incidence of which remains high. According to data from the World Health Organisation, out of 50 million deaths worldwide each year, ischaemic heart disease is the leading cause of death, with 7.4 million deaths due to coronary heart disease. [1]. In Algeria, its prognosis remains serious, with MI still responsible for 8% of total annual mortality in adults [[2]. To this mortality must be added a significant morbidity and the socio-economic repercussions that it represents.

Despite remarkable advances in the treatment of MI, diagnosis in the emergency department remains a complex clinical problem. [[3, 4]. Although the physician's clinical impression is a very sensitive indicator of MI, between 4% and 11.8% of patients presenting to the emergency department with MI will be undiagnosed and discharged from hospital without treatment [5, 6]. Similarly, more than 80% of patients admitted to coronary care units following indications suggestive of MI will be discharged without being able to confirm a diagnosis of infarction [7, 8].

As the majority of cardiac deaths occur in the pre-hospital phase [[9-11]early detection of the first symptoms of ischaemic heart disease would most likely lead to better and, consequently, more appropriate treatment, improve patients' quality of life and reduce the cost to society. Several epidemiological studies have demonstrated the potential impact in terms of mortality and cardiac morbidity of a reduction in the time between the onset of symptoms and the effective management of patients [11, 12]. In practice, this time should be reduced to less than two hours, compared with the current average of four hours [[11, 13-15]. But the problem is not a simple one; even the best experts are sometimes wrong. In addition, cardiac ischaemia can be unstable: present at the patient's home, it may disappear on arrival at the emergency department, only to reappear a few hours later when the patient has returned home; hence the interest in infarct prediction solutions.

A number of approaches have been proposed to improve the relevance of the diagnosis of MI by clinicians [16-21]]. These approaches based on diagnostic algorithms have been developed using logistic regression and the latter is based on linear models and the practical success of its approach is limited by its linearity [22]. To date, none of these approaches has been widely adopted. It has been suggested that doctors will only use a method that aims to improve diagnostic accuracy if it is easy to use and significantly and consistently improves their performance [23, 24][.

In recent years, the use of artificial neural networks (ANNs) has developed in a number of disciplines, particularly in medicine. They are mainly used to solve classification and prediction problems [25]. In the context of data processing, ANNs are a method of approximating complex systems, particularly useful when these systems are difficult to model using conventional statistical methods such as logistic regression. ANNs are also applicable in all situations where there is a non-linear relationship between a predictor variable and a predicted variable [26].

As a linear association between the variables associated with MI cannot be assumed, which is required by other statistical analyses, a RNA could help predict MI and could even exceed the performance of the regression analysis usually applied.

This work has two objectives:

The first objective is to develop, using artificial neural networks and logistic regression, two models for predicting MI based on data available at the time of presentation of patients to cardiology emergency departments at the University Hospital Establishment (EHU) in Oran.

2. Methods

2.1. Type of study

This is a comparative study of two prediction models for MI. The study was conducted in the cardiology emergency department of the EHU of Oran, Algeria, between January 2015 and December 2015.

2.2. Study population

The study involved all patients who presented to the cardiology emergency department of the EHU of Oran with chest pain as the reason for referral.

2.2.1. Case definition

The diagnosis of MI was based on the presence of at least two of the following criteria [[27]:

1- Clinical: intense angina pain lasting more than 30 minutes.
2- Electrical (signs present in at least two concordant leads of the standard ECG): development and persistence of new Q waves or QS waves of duration $\geq$ 0.04 s; decrease in R waves of at least 25%; change in ST segment and/or T waves suggestive of transmural ischaemia.
3- Enzymatic: elevation of troponin.

The type of MI was classified with or without ST-segment elevation, as defined in the universal classification [28].

2.2.2. Inclusion criteria

Patients over the age of 18 consulting an emergency department for chest pain were included in the study.

2.2.3. Exclusion criteria

Patients with chest pain of traumatic origin.

2.2.4. Judging criteria

The endpoint was the evaluation of the diagnostic performance of the predictive models developed by the neural logistic approach in the diagnosis of MI. Diagnostic performance was measured using ROC curves (Receiver Operating Curve).

2.2.5. Sample size

For the model to be considered useful, we based ourselves on its sensitivity in detecting pathology. This is the sensitivity of the predictive model to identify MI among patients consulting for chest pain.

The sample size required to demonstrate the clinical utility of the diagnostic algorithm was estimated as follows. To detect MI, our analysis should focus on sensitivity (Se), to ensure the lowest possible false-negative rate (1-Se). To be of clinical interest, our rule should have a sensitivity of at least 80%. The predictive model would be considered ineffective if we were unable to obtain a model with a sensitivity of at least 73%. [29]which corresponds approximately to clinicians' performance in ruling out the diagnosis of MI. Assuming an average rate of MI of 25 [30][the number of subjects required is calculated according to the following formula [[31]:

$$N = \frac{\varepsilon^2 Se(1 - Se)}{d^2 \text{ x p}}$$

Where:

- N: sample size.

- ε: parameter related to the accepted statistical risk of error (here, equal to 1.96 for a 5% risk of error).
- Se: sensitivity of our diagnostic algorithm (80%).
- p: the proportion of patients presenting to the cardiac emergency department with chest pain who have MI (according to Eggers et al. [[30]it is 25%).
- d: sensitivity accuracy (80% - 73% = 7%).

The inclusion of 502 patients with chest pain would ensure the usefulness of our predictive model.

2.2.6. Patient recruitment

This study involved all patients admitted for chest pain to the cardiology emergency department of the EHU of Oran between January 2015 and December 2015.

2.2.7. Conduct of the study

Patients admitted to the emergency department with chest pain underwent guided medical observation in the form of questioning, clinical examination, requests for further tests and specialist advice. Demographic and clinical data, cardiovascular risk factors, electrocardiographic appearance on admission and results of cardiac biomarkers were collected for all patients.

All patients with a presumptive diagnosis of MI were admitted to a cardiac intensive care unit and followed until discharge.

2.3. Data collection

The survey was conducted using a three-part questionnaire:

The first stage involved patient identification:

1. Patient identity.

2. Sex.

3. Age.

The second part dealt with the clinical aspects of the patient:

4. The concept of smoking has been defined in three categories: a current smoker is someone who has smoked in the previous 12 months, a former smoker is someone who has stopped smoking for more than a year, and a non-smoker is someone who has never smoked. [32].

5. Personal history of hypertension, diabetes and dyslipidaemia.

6. Personal and family history of coronary heart disease.

7. The time between the onset of symptoms and admission to the emergency department was defined by three classes: less than 6 hours, 6 to 12 hours and more than 12 hours. [19].

8. Measurement of blood pressure (systolic and diastolic): blood pressure is considered high if systolic pressure is $\geq$ 140 mmHg and/or diastolic pressure is $\geq$ 90 mmHg; it is considered low if systolic pressure is $\leq$ 90 mmHg and/or diastolic pressure is $\leq$ 50 mmHg [33].

9. Measurement of heart rate (HR): heart rate was considered high if it was $\geq$ 100 bpm and considered low if it was $\leq$ 50 bpm [33][.

10. There are four Killip scores: stage 1 is considered when there is no sign of heart failure, stage 2 when there is moderate heart failure, stage 3 when there is frank pulmonary oedema and stage 4 when there is cardiogenic shock or hypotension. [34].

The third section looked at ECG tracing data for :

11. Sus ST segment shift.

12. ST segment undershoot.

13. Necrosis Q wave.

2.4. Statistical analysis and comparison of predictive models

2.4.1. Linear trend test

To test the linear trend of the associations with the quantitative exposure variables, we generated a continuous variable taking the median value of each class of categorical variables for each subject in that class. The deviation from linearity was then tested by a maximum likelihood test comparing the model containing this quantitative variable with the model containing the categorical variable. If the linearity hypothesis was not rejected, the linear trend was tested by the deviation from 0 of the slope associated with the quantitative variable.

2.4.2. Artificial neural network

The RNA used in this study is the multilayer backpropagation perceptron [35] with IDM as output variable.

The backpropagation algorithm calculates the mean square error, which measures the error between the output provided by the network and the desired output. Given a set of examples which are pairs (inputs, desired outputs), the network is first initialised, i.e. the synaptic weights are given randomly to allow the network to start learning. At each stage, an example is presented as input and the network calculates an output. The error is then calculated by comparing the calculated output with the expected output. This error is then backpropagated in the network, resulting in a modification of each weight that contributed to the error. This process is repeated, presenting each example in turn. The learning process consists of minimising the mean square error for all the examples.

To reduce the data sample size and determine the optimal set of input variables, qualified network sensitivity analyses were performed primarily to prioritise variables in the data set [36]. In detail, this method examines each available input variable using a neural network. For each variable removed from the input list, the mean square error of the output is calculated. Only those variables that result in a deterioration in model performance by being dropped are retained in the final architecture of the network. The lower the error, the better the performance of the network.

Given that neural network models are built by learning from a certain number of observations, the patient data was randomly divided into training and test series. We used 70% of the observations (378 patients) for training (learning) and 30% for testing (162 patients), in order to test the real predictive capacity of the network. In order to avoid over-training the network, a validation base of 108 patients taken from the training base was used to interrupt the process of modifying the weights of the neural network when the validation error left its minimum.

2.4.3. Logistic regression

Binary logistic regression [37] was used to predict MDI. In order to identify the variables used in the logistic model, a univariate analysis was performed and the variables at the 20% significance level were retained for the final model. Interactions between variables were tested using a likelihood test at the 10% significance level. Finally, the variables used to design the predictive model were selected using a stepwise top-down strategy at the 5% level. The model was built on the basis of the training data and tested on the observations of the test group.

A clinical score predictive of MI was constructed. This score was derived by rounding the β_i coefficients associated with each predictor to a whole number. To ensure that there was no difference between the roundings and the original logistic regression model, their areas under the ROC curve were compared.

2.4.4. Model calibration

For each model, the fit was checked using the Hosmer-Lemeshow Chi² test [37]. A model is well calibrated when the predicted probabilities of the model are not statistically significantly different (p > 0.05) from the observed frequencies.

In this study, patients were divided into decile of probability predicted by the models, and a Chi² test with 8 degrees of freedom was performed between the number of patients expected by the predicted probability and the observed number of patients in each decile.

2.4.5. Model comparison

The comparison between RNA and binary logistic regression was made by analysing their ROC curves. In the ROC analysis, diagnostic performance (prediction of MI) is reported in terms of two indices, namely the true-positive fraction (sensitivity) and the false-positive fraction (1-specificity). The area under the curve (AUC) was calculated using the method of Hanley and McNeil [38]and the ROC curves were compared using the method of DeLong et al. [39].

The correct classification rate (CCR), sensitivity, specificity, positive predictive value (PPV) and negative predictive value (NPV) of each model were calculated from the confusion matrices.

2.4.6. Statistics

Qualitative variables were expressed as percentages and quantitative variables as averages. The Chi² test was used to compare percentages and the Student's *t-test* to compare means at the 5% significance level.

The RNA was calculated using SAS JMP Pro version 10. Logistic regression was performed with SPSS version 20. ROC curves were constructed and compared using Stata SE version 12 software.

2.5. Ethical considerations

Our study was carried out on patients' files and ethical aspects were respected, given that the confidentiality of patients' data was ensured.

3. Results

3.1. Description of the total study population

3.1.1. Age and sex

Our survey included 540 patients admitted to cardiology emergency departments with non-traumatic chest pain. There were 294 men (54.4%) and 246 women (45.6%), giving a sex ratio of 1.2 (Fig. 1).

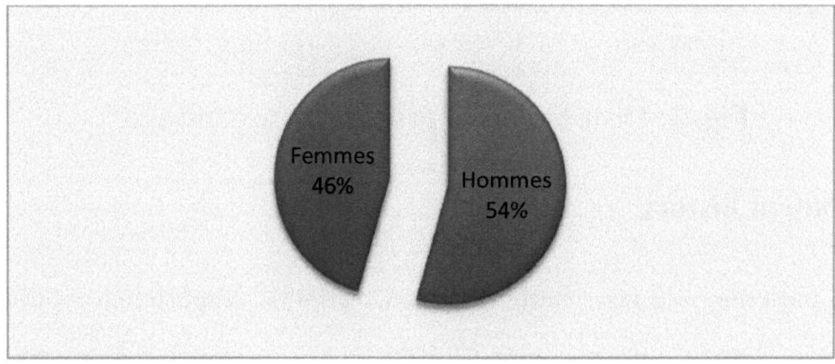

Fig. 1: Breakdown of the total study population by gender.

The mean age of the patients was 57.1 ± 12.3 years, with extremes ranging from 24 to 92 years. The mean age did not differ significantly by sex, being 57.1 ± 12.4 years in men and 56.4 ± 12.2 years in women (p = 0.226) (Table 1).

Table 1. Age of patients admitted to emergency departments with chest pain.

	Average (years)	Standard deviation	p
Total population	57,1	12,3	
Men	57,1	12,4	0,266
Women	56,4	12,2	

The age distribution of the sample was as follows: 18.1% of patients were under 45, 56.1% between 45 and 65 and 25.7% over 65. In terms of gender, the

45-65 age group was the most represented (55.8% for men and 56.5% for women) (Fig. 2).

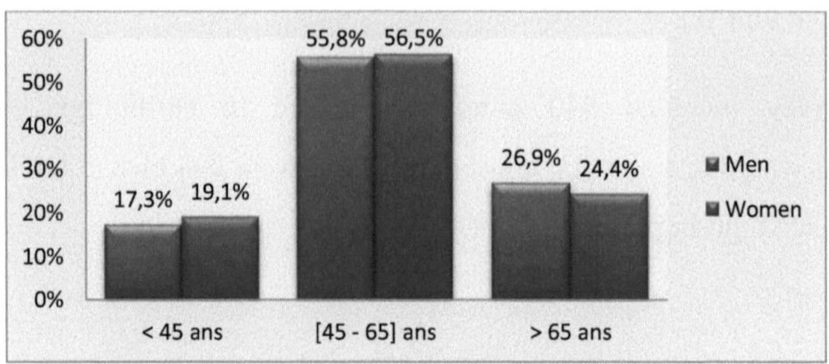

Fig. 2: Distribution of patients by sex and age.

3.1.2. Patient history

Of all patients, 22.6% had diabetes, 29.4% hypertension and 17.4% dyslipidaemia. Thirty-nine patients (7.2%) had a personal history of coronary heart disease and 18.3% of patients had a family history of coronary heart disease (Fig. 3).

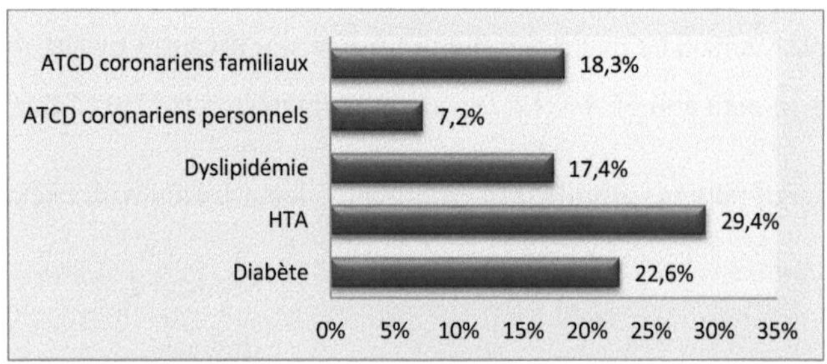

Fig. 3: Distribution of patients according to cardiovascular history.

3.1.3. Tobacco consumption

Former smokers accounted for 11.9% of our study population, while 12.8% of patients still smoked (Fig. 4). Current smoking was reported by 21.4% of men and 2.43% of women ($p < 10^{-3}$) (Table 2).

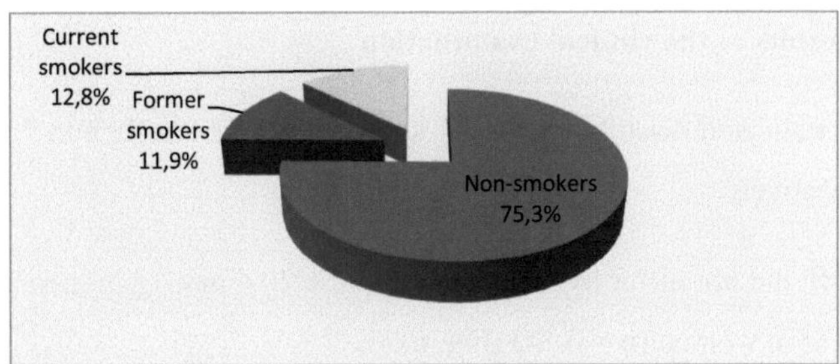

Fig. 4: Distribution of patients according to smoking status.

Table 2. Breakdown of patients by sex and smoking status.

	Men		Woman	
	n	**%**	**n**	**%**
Non-smokers	171	58,2	236	95,9
Former smokers	60	20,4	4	1,6
Current smokers	63	21,4	6	2,4

3.1.4. Emergency call times

The average admission time (onset of symptoms - arrival at hospital) was 36 ± 22 hours (range 1 to 445 hours). Two hundred patients (36.9%) arrived before 6 hours and 210 patients (38.8%) were admitted after 12 hours of pain onset (Fig. 5).

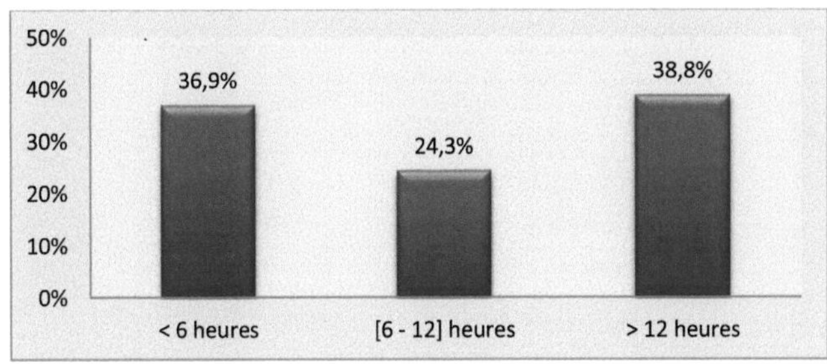

Fig. 5: Distribution of patients by time from onset of pain to admission.

3.1.5. Results of the clinical examination

Mean systolic and diastolic pressures were 129 ± 19.7 mmHg and 75.1 ± 12.7 mmHg respectively.

Mean SBP did not differ by sex, being 130.2 ± 20.4 mmHg in men and 127.7 ± 18.9 mmHg in women (p = 0.14) (Fig. 6).

Also, no difference was found between mean DBP and sex (p = 0.926). The mean DBP for men was 75.1 ± 12.6 mmHg and for women 75.2 ± 12.7 mmHg (Fig. 7).

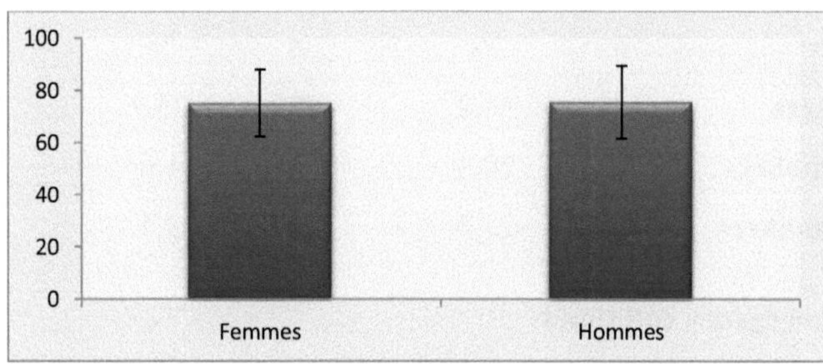

Fig. 6: Distribution of systolic blood pressure in men and women.

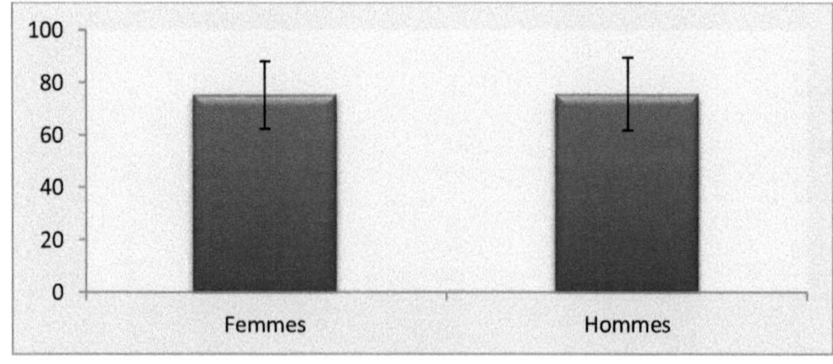

Fig. 7: Distribution of diastolic blood pressure in men and women.

On admission, four patients (0.7%) had low blood pressure, 375 patients (69.4%) had normal blood pressure and 161 patients (29.8%) had high blood pressure (Fig. 8).

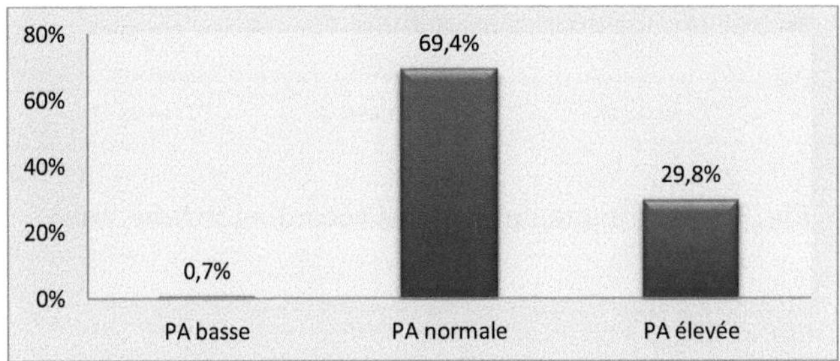

Fig. 8: Distribution of patients according to blood pressure.

The mean heart rate was 75.5 ± 13.4 bpm. It was 75.6 ± 13.9 bpm in men and 75.2 ± 12.8 bpm in women (p = 0.709) (Fig. 9).

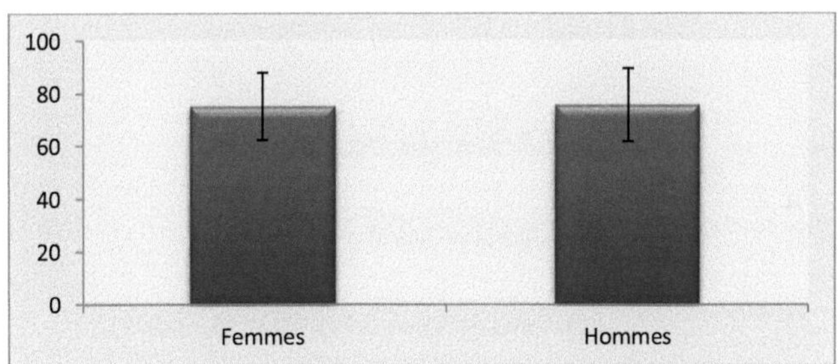

Fig. 9: Distribution of heart rate by sex.

Heart rate was low in 1.9%, normal in 94.6% and high in 3.5% (Fig. 10).

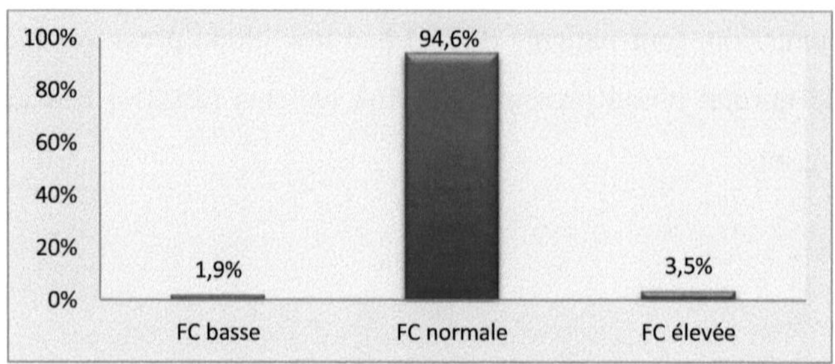

Fig. 10: Distribution of patients according to heart rate.

3.1.6. Electrocardiographic results

In terms of ECG data, 31.3% of patients had ST-segment elevation, 15.4% of patients had ST-segment undershift and 20.9% of patients had a Q wave (Fig. 11).

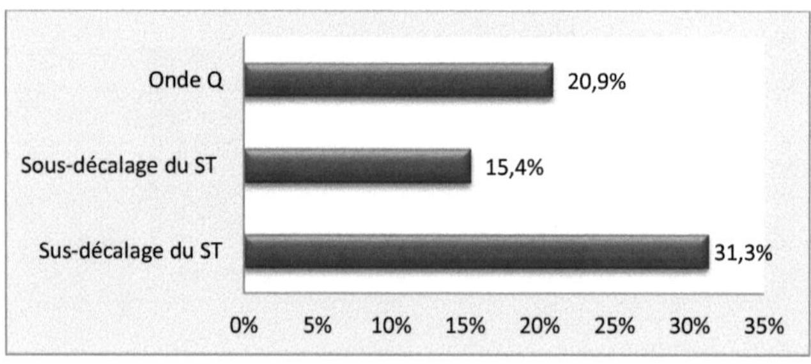

Fig. 11 Distribution of patients according to ECG results.

3.2. Profile of patients with MI

3.2.1. Age and sex

During the study period, 118 patients had presented with MI on admission, representing a proportion of 21.8% (26.2% in men vs. 16.7% in women, p = 0.008). There were 77 men (65.3%) and 41 women (34.7%), giving a sex ratio of 1.9 (Fig. 12).

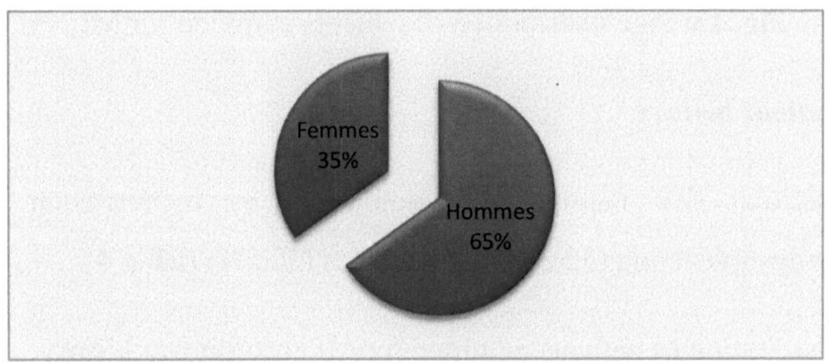

Fig. 12 Distribution of patients admitted for MI by sex.

The mean age was 58.9 ± 12.3 years (Table 3). It was 58 ± 11.9 years in men and 60.7 ± 13.1 years in women (p = 0.277).

Table 3. Age of patients admitted for MI.

	Average (years)	Standard deviation	p
Population admitted for MI	58,9	12,3	
Men	58	11,9	0,277
Women	60,7	13,1	

The most representative age group was between 45 and 65 (57.6%), followed by patients aged over 65 (28%) (Fig. 13).

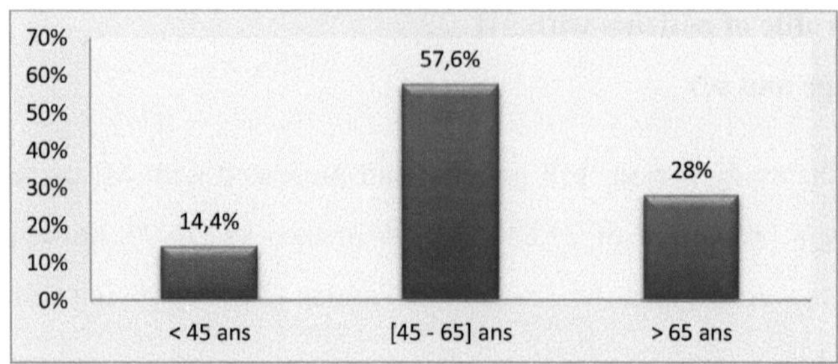

Fig. 13: Age distribution of patients admitted for MI.

3.2.2. Patient history

Cardiovascular risk factors were dominated by hypertension (41.5%), followed by dyslipidaemia (32.2%) and diabetes (30.5%) (table 4).

Table 4. Distribution of patients admitted for MI according to history.

History	n	%
Diabetes		
No	82	69,5
Yes	36	30,5
HTA		
No	69	58,5
Yes	49	41,5
Dyslipidemia		
No	80	67,8
Yes	38	32,2
Personal history of coronary heart disease	103	87,3
No	15	12,7
Yes		

Family history of coronary heart disease		
No	97	82,2
Yes	21	17,8

3.2.3. Tobacco consumption

Smoking was reported in 29.8% of men and 7.4% of women ($p < 10^{-3}$) (table 5).

Table 5. Breakdown of patients by sex and smoking status.

	Men		Woman		Total	
	n	**%**	**n**	**%**	**n**	**%**
Non-smokers	33	42,9	37	90,2	70	59,4
Former smokers	21	27,3	1	2,4	22	18,6
Current smokers	23	29,8	3	7,4	26	22

Patients under 65 were the main smokers. Smoking accounted for 23.5% of patients aged under 45, rising to 27.9% of patients aged between 45 and 65 (Fig. 14).

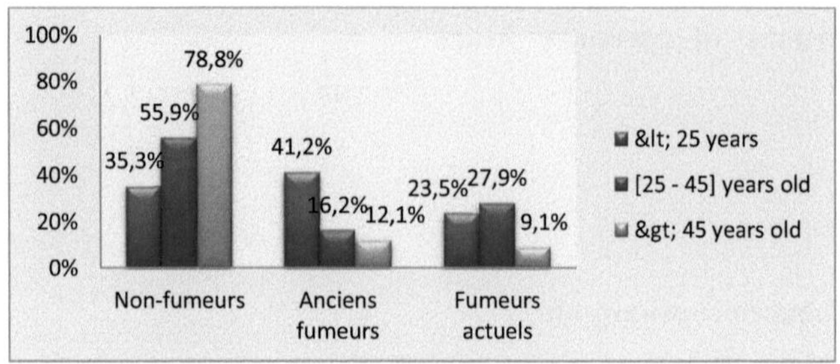

Fig. 14: Distribution of patients admitted for MI by age and smoking status.

3.2.4. Emergency call times

The average arrival time was 26.33 ± 21.3 hours (range 1 to 320 hours). Half of the patients (59 patients) with MI were seen within the first 6 hours (Fig. 15).

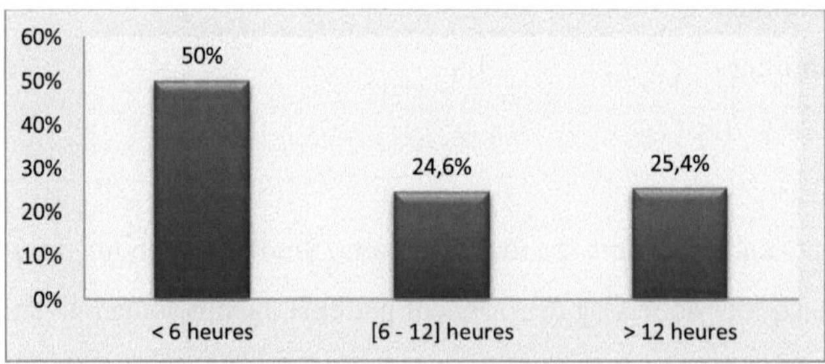

Fig. 15: Distribution of patients admitted for MI according to the time between onset of pain and admission.

3.2.5. Results of the clinical examination

On admission, mean SBP was 129.3 ± 24.6 mmHg, mean DBP was 76.2 ± 14.8 mmHg and mean heart rate was 83.2 ± 19.3 mmHg. Blood pressure and heart rate were normal at 71.2% and 84.7% respectively. Eighty-three patients (70.4%) were admitted as Killip stage 1 and 32 patients (27.2%) as Killip stage 2 (table 6).

Table 6. Distribution of patients admitted for MI according to clinical examination.

Characteristics of the clinical examination	n	%
Blood pressure		
Low	3	2,5
Normal	84	71,2
High	31	26,3
Heart rate		
Low	4	3,4
Normal	100	84,7
High	14	11,9
Killip score		
Killip 1	83	70,4
Killip 2	32	27,2
Killip 3	2	1,6
Killip 4	1	0,8

3.2.6. Electrocardiographic results

From an electrocardiographic point of view, ST elevation was observed in 71 patients (60.2%) and ST sub-shift in 26 patients (22%). Seventy-one patients (60.2%) progressed to Q-wave MI and 47 (39.8%) to non-Q-wave MI (Fig. 16).

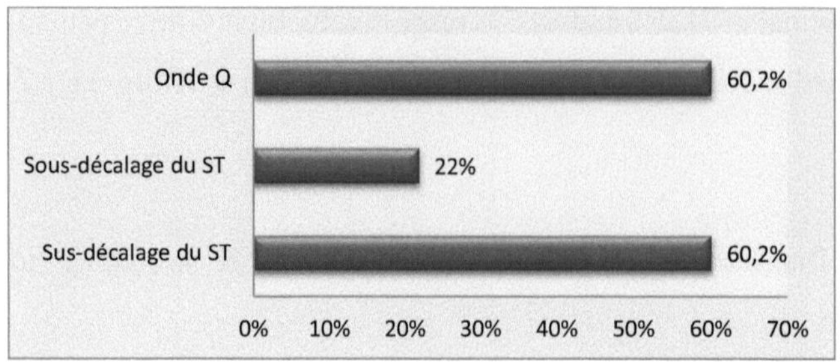

Fig. 16 Distribution of patients admitted for MI according to ECG tracing results.

The electrocardiogram showed anterior infarction (50%), posterior infarction (30.5%), lateral infarction (11.8%), deep septal infarction (4.2%) and circumferential infarction (3.4%). Table 7 shows the topography of ECG abnormalities during MI.

Table 7. Topographical diagnosis of MI.

Territory	n	%
Previous	59	50
Posterior	36	30,5
Lateral	14	11,8
Deep septal vein	5	4,2
Circumferential	4	3,4

3.3. Statistical analysis of results

3.3.1. Linear trend test

The linearity test was non-significant for the variables age (p = 0.986), DBP (p = 0.411), SBP (p = 830), and heart rate (p = 0.061). As a result, all of the above variables were retained in quantitative form.

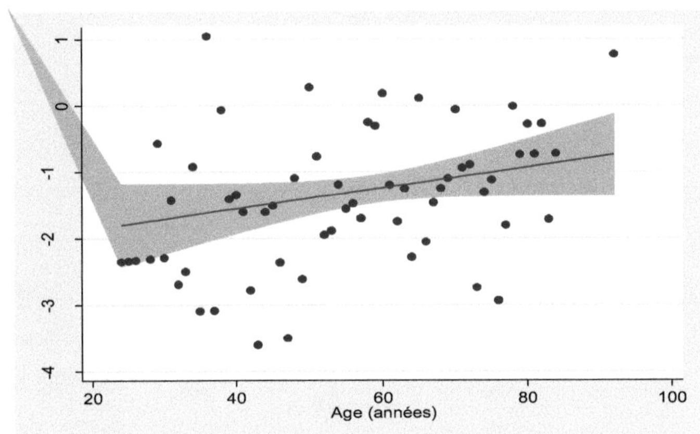

Fig. 17: Modelling of the "age" variable (p = 0.986).

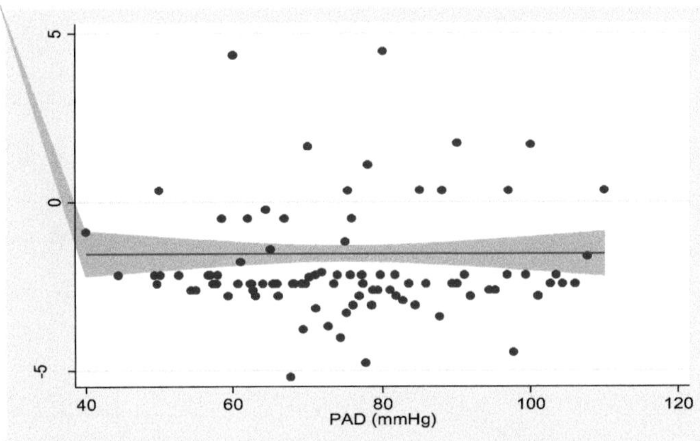

Fig. 18 Modelling of the "diastolic blood pressure" variable (p = 0.411).

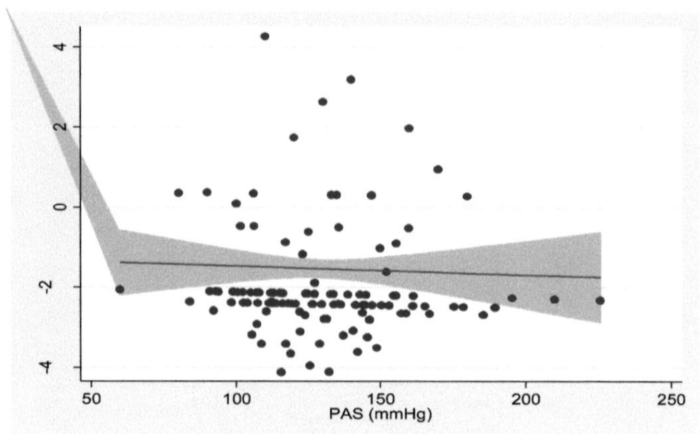

Fig. 19 Modelling of the "systolic blood pressure" variable (p = 830).

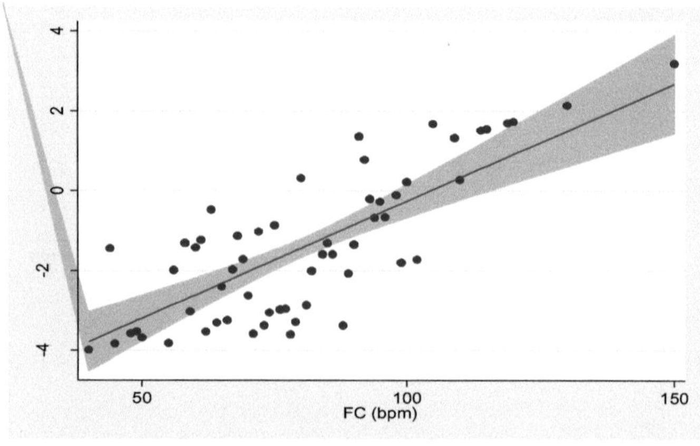

Fig. 20: Modelling of the "heart rate" variable (p = 0.061).

However, the maximum likelihood test showed that the variable "time between onset of pain and admission to emergency" deviated significantly from linearity (p = 0.001) and this variable was introduced into the predictive model as being discrete (less than 6 hours, between 6 and 12 hours, and greater than 12 hours).

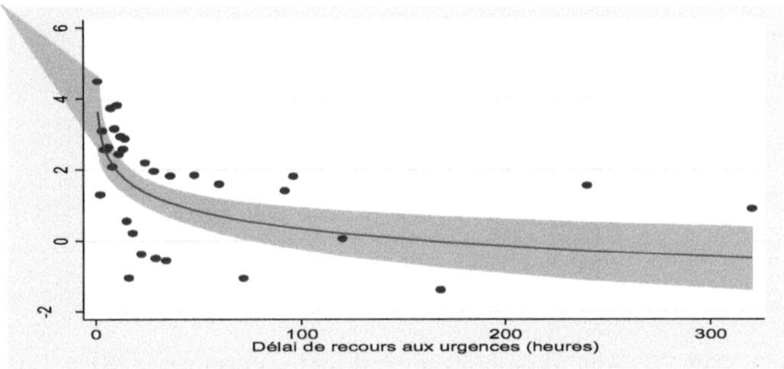

Fig. 21: Modelling of the variable "time taken to use emergency services" (p = 0.001).

3.3.2. Comparison of the characteristics of MI versus non-MI patients
3.3.2.1. Comparison by gender

The proportion of men was significantly higher in patients with MI than in patients without MI (65.3% vs. 51.4%; p = 0.008) (Fig. 22).

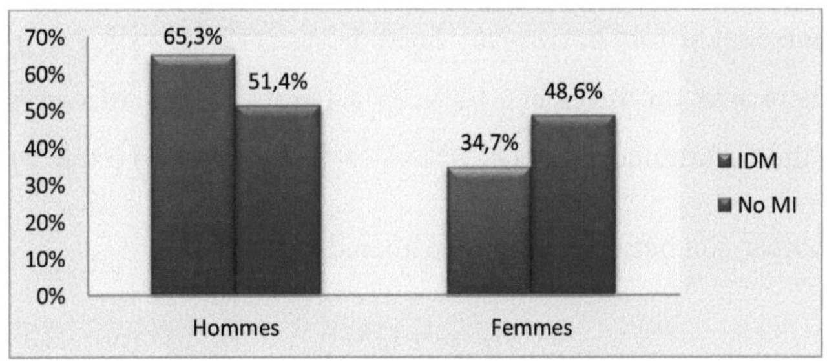

Fig. 22. Distribution of patients by sex and presence of MI.

3.3.2.2. Comparison by age

The mean age did not differ significantly (p = 0.069) between the group of patients diagnosed with MI (58.9 ± 12.3 years) and the group of patients with chest pain without MI (56.6 ± 12.3 years) (Fig. 23).

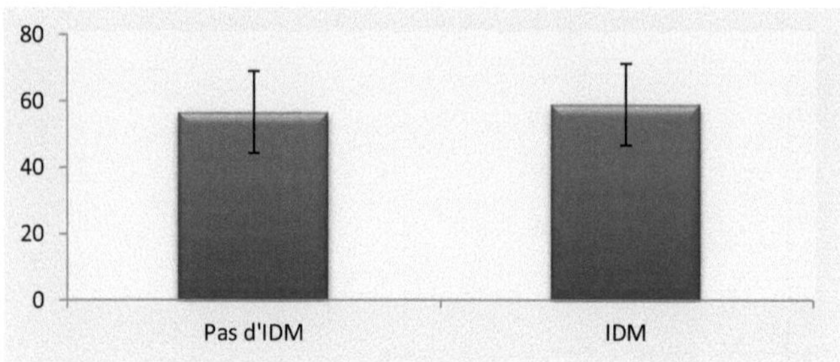

Fig. 23. Age of patients according to presence of MI.

3.3.2.3. Comparison by patient history

MI was significantly associated with diabetes (30.5% vs 20.4%; p = 0.02), hypertension (41.5% vs 26.1%; p = 0.001), dyslipidaemia (32.2% vs 13.3%; p < 0.001) and personal history of coronary heart disease (12.7% vs 5.7%; p = 0.009). 10^{-3}) and personal history of coronary heart disease (12.7% vs 5.7%; p = 0.009). However, there was no difference between a family history of coronary heart disease and the occurrence of MI (17.8% vs 18.5%; p = 0.865) (table 8).

Table 8. Comparison between patients with and without MI.

Variables	MI (n = 118)		No MI (n = 422)		p
	n	%	n	%	
Diabetes					0,020

No	82	69,5	336	79,6	
Yes	36	30,5	86	20,4	
HTA					0,001
No	69	58,5	312	73,9	
Yes	49	41,5	110	26,1	
Dyslipidemia					$< 10^{-3}$
No	80	67,8	366	86,7	
Yes	38	32,2	56	13,3	
Personal history of coronary heart disease					0,009
No	103	87,3	398	94,3	
Yes	15	12,7	24	5,7	
Family history of coronary heart disease					0,865
No	97	82,2	344	81,5	
Yes	21	17,8	78	18,5	

A statistically significant relationship was also found between smoking and the onset of MI. The frequency of former smokers in patients with MI was 18.6% compared with 10% in patients without MI (p = 0.011). Also, current smokers were significantly more numerous in patients with MI (22% vs 10.2%; $p < 10^{-3}$) (Fig. 24).

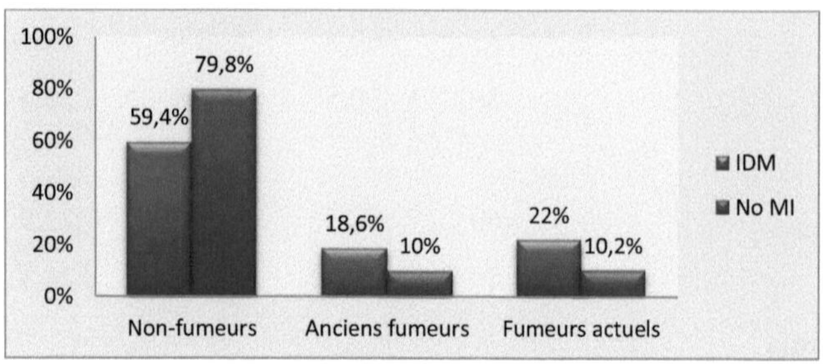

Fig. 24: Distribution of patients by smoking status and presence of MI.

3.3.2.4. Comparison by clinical examination

Mean SBP and mean DBP did not differ significantly between the MI and non-MI groups. However, mean heart rate was significantly higher in patients with MI (83.2 bpm vs 73.3 bpm; $p < 10^{-3}$) (table 9).

Table 9. Comparison between patients with and without MI according to clinical parameters.

Variables	MI (n = 118)		No MI (n = 422)		p
	Average	AND	Average	AND	
Systolic blood pressure	129,3	24,6	129	18,2	0,881
Diastolic blood pressure	76,2	14,8	74,8	12	0,317
Heart rate	83,2	19,3	73,3	10,3	$< 10^{-3}$

A statistically significant relationship was found between the duration of symptoms and the presence of MI. The percentage of MI was higher when the time between the onset of symptoms and admission to emergency was less than 6 hours (50% vs. 33.2%; p = 0.001) (Fig. 25).

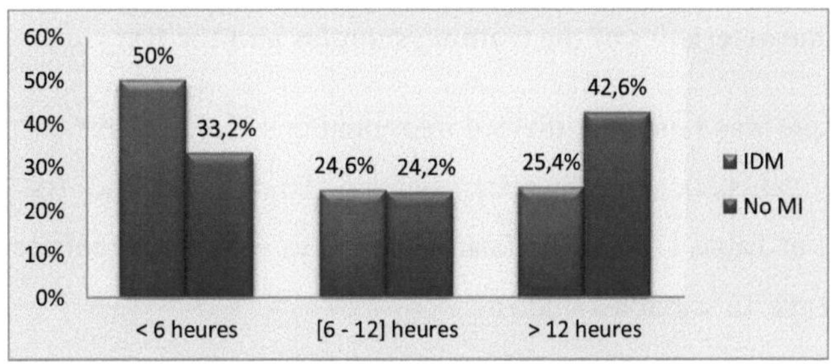

Fig. 25. Distribution of patients according to duration of symptoms and presence of MI.

3.3.2.5. Comparison according to electrocardiographic results

The onset of MI was significantly associated with ST-segment elevation (60.2% vs 23.2%; $p < 10^{-3}$), ST-segment sub-shift (22% vs 13.5%; p = 0.023) and the appearance of a Q wave on the ECG tracing (60.2% vs 10%; $p < 10^{-3}$) (table 10).

Table 10. Comparison between patients with and without MI according to ECG data.

Variables	MI (n = 118)		No MI (n = 422)		p
	n	%	n	%	
ST segment elevation					$< 10^{-3}$
No	47	39,8	324	76,8	
Yes	71	60,2	98	23,2	
ST segment sub-shift					0,023
No	92	78,0	365	86,5	
Yes	26	22,0	57	13,5	
Q wave					$< 10^{-3}$
No	47	39,8	380	90,0	
Yes	71	60,2	42	10,0	

3.3.3. Characteristics of the training samples and the test

Our sample was randomly divided into training series (378 patients) and test series (162 patients). The characteristics of the training and test data are summarised in Table 11. No significant differences were found between the two data sets for the 15 variables studied.

Table 11. Comparison of training and test data.

Variables	Learning	Test	p
Age	$56,9 \pm 11,9$	$57,6 \pm 13,4$	0,555
Gender			0,598
Male	203 (53,7%)	91 (56,2%)	
Female	175 (46,3%)	71 (43,8%)	
Diabetes			0,59
No	295 (75,9%)	123 (78%)	
Yes	83 (24,1%)	39 (22%)	
HTA			0,578
No	264 (69,8%)	117 (72,2%)	
Yes	114 (30,2%)	45 (27,8%)	
Dyslipidemia			0,235
No	317 (83,9%)	129 (79,6%)	
Yes	61 (16,1%)	33 (20,4%)	
Personal history of coronary heart disease			0,80
No	350 (92,6%)	151 (93,2%)	
Yes	28 (7,4%)	11 (6,8%)	
Family history of coronary heart disease			0,297
No	313 (82,8%)	128 (79%)	
	65 (17,2%)	34 (21%)	

Yes		
Tobacco consumption		0,21
Non-smokers	288 (76,2%)	119 (73,5%)
Former smokers	39 (10,3%)	25 (15,4%)
Current smokers	51 (13,5%)	18 (11,1%)

Table 11 (continued)

Variables	Learning	Test	p
Duration of symptoms			0,461
< 6 hours	133 (35,2%)	66 (40,7%)	
Between 6 and 12 hours	95 (25,1%)	36 (22,3%)	
> 12 **hours**	150 (39,7%)	60 (37%)	
NO*T*	129,2 ± 19,7	128,9 ± 19,7	0,865
PAD	74,6 ± 14,8	74,8 ± 12	0,317
Heart rate	74,5 ± 12,9	77,1 ± 14,4	0,063
ST elevation			0,504
No	263 (69,6%)	108 (66,7%)	
Yes	115 (30,4%)	54 (33,3%)	
ST sub-shift			0,112
No	326 (86,2%)	131 (80,9%)	
Yes	52 (13,8%)	31 (19,1%)	
Q wave			0,503
No	296 (78,3%)	131 (80,9%)	
Yes	82 (21,7%)	31 (19,1%)	

3.3.4. Predictive analysis

3.3.4.1. Artificial neural network analysis

The architecture of the network used in this study is illustrated in Figure 26. The network was composed of three layers: an input layer, a hidden layer and an output layer.

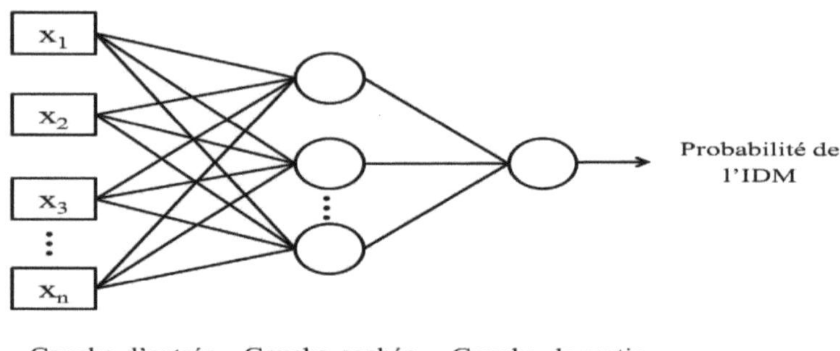

Fig. 26. Architecture of the neural network.

The best configuration in terms of the architecture of the neural networks used for IDM prediction was determined experimentally by training h x n x t structures obtained by setting the number of hidden layers to a single layer (h = 1) and varying the number of neurons in the hidden layer (n = 5, 6, 7, ..., 15) and the type of activation function (t = linear, sigmoid, tangent-sigmoid).

The detailed performance results of the h x n x t structures in terms of mean square error (MSE) are shown in Table 1

Table 12. Summary of neural network performance results.

Number of neurons in the hidden layer	Activation functions	MSE of the learning sample	MSE of the test sample
5	linear	0,312	0,322
6	linear	0,336	0,352
7	linear	0,355	0,361
8	linear	0,329	0,338
9	linear	0,403	0,418
10	linear	0,356	0,378
11	linear	0,376	0,389
12	linear	0,345	0,360
13	linear	0,338	0,352
14	linear	0,378	0,388
15	linear	0,398	0,409
5	sigmoid	0,332	0,338
6	sigmoid	0,345	0,351
7	sigmoid	0,321	0,342
8	sigmoid	0,356	0,375
9	sigmoid	0,367	0,379
10	sigmoid	0,354	0,376
11	sigmoid	0,325	0,335
12	sigmoid	0,371	0,381
13	sigmoid	0,376	0,378
14	sigmoid	0,378	0,389
15	sigmoid	0,403	0,409
5	tangent-sigmoid	0,312	0,324
6	tangent-sigmoid	0,298	0,301

7	**tangent-sigmoid**	**0,266**	**0,269**
8	tangent-sigmoid	0,278	0,290
9	tangent-sigmoid	0,289	0,302
10	tangent-sigmoid	0,389	0,403

Table 12 (continued)

Number of neurons in the hidden layer	Activation functions	MSE of the learning sample	MSE of the test sample
11	tangent-sigmoid	0,304	0,326
12	tangent-sigmoid	0,298	0,317
13	tangent-sigmoid	0,297	0,315
14	tangent-sigmoid	0,305	0,330
15	tangent-sigmoid	0,308	0,314

Table 13 shows that the optimal number of neurons in the hidden layer is 7 with a tangent-sigmoid activation function. This network gave us the lowest mean square error for both the training and test samples, which were 0.266 and 0.269 respectively.

The sensitivity of the variables used in the neural model is summarised in Table 17. The errors were compared with the baseline error of 0.266. Six variables (gender, diabetes, family history of coronary heart disease, duration of symptoms, SBP and DBP) were found to degrade the model.

As a result, the input layer of the network was composed of nine input neurons (age, hypertension, dyslipidaemia, personal coronary history, smoking status, heart rate, ST elevation, ST sub-shift and Q wave), the hidden layer was composed of seven neurons with a tangent-sigmoid activation function and the output layer was composed of one output neuron with a sigmoid activation function (Fig. 27).

Table 13. Sensitivity analysis of input variables.

Input variables	Error after deletion
Age	0,285
Gender	0,260
Diabetes	0,260
HTA	0,271
Dyslipidemia	0,275
Personal history of coronary heart disease	0,267
Family history of coronary heart disease	0,261
Smoking status	0,271
Duration of symptoms	0,265
NOT	0,238
PAD	0,252
Heart rate	0,284
ST elevation	0,281
ST sub-shift	0,268
Q wave	0,308

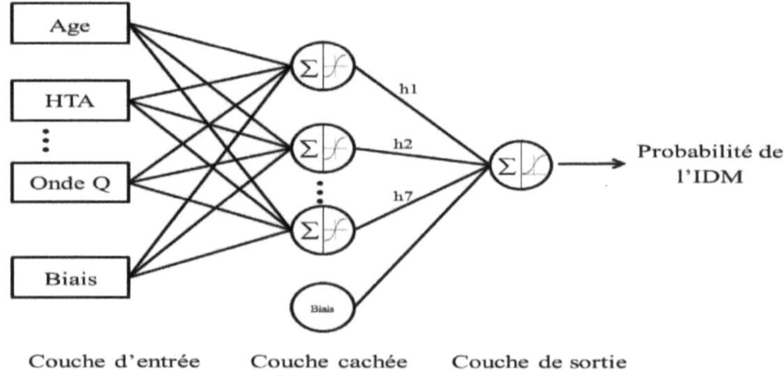

Fig. 27. Architecture of the neural network for diagnosing MDI.

Table 14 gives the synaptic weights of the multilayer perceptron used for IDM prediction. These coefficients represent the connections between the seven hidden layer neurons (h1, ..., h7) and all the input neurons.

Table 14. Input layer synaptic weights.

Variables	h1	h2	h3	h4	h5	h6	h7
Age	0,001286	0,005946	0,02182	0,019058	0,022109	0,00558	-0,0423
HTA	-0,53776	0,99226	0,642945	0,03336	0,048452	0,10124	0,02713
Dyslipidemia	0,469631	0,194498	0,23755	0,408117	0,17321	0,58622	0,31005
Personal history of coronary	0,81086	1,82473	2,11179	0,976973	0,99473	-0,4927	1,035461

heart disease						
Tobacco consumption	-0,00402	-0,14336	0,294542	-0,64644	-0,34212	-0,67523	0,108493
Heart rate	0,000552	0,012145	0,028881	-0,00688	-0,01353	-0,03798	0,007771
ST elevation	-0,65046	0,564055	0,580157	-0,55495	-0,61382	-1,0432	0,009063
ST offset	0,192241	-0,57649	-0,017655	1,210602	0,667809	-0,81258	-0,66893
Q wave	0,111617	0,419856	0,742007	-1,29188	0,221202	-2,01517	0,2639
Bias	0,222337	-1,8099	-4,85774	0,608589	0,515256	6,366217	1,51612

At each hidden node, a weighted linear combination of the inputs is summed, then a tangent-sigmoid transformation is applied.

The weights linking the hidden layer and the output neuron are shown in Table 15.

Table 15. Hidden layer synaptic weights.

Hidden neurons	Coefficients
h1	-0,12829
h2	0,07448
h3	0,0584
h4	0,15043
h5	0,039864
h6	-0,59325
h7	0,047955
Bias	0,49511

The probability of having the IDM = 1/ [1+exp -($bias + \Sigma h_i$ $hidden$ $node_i$)]

The neural predictive model showed good calibration (Hosmer-Lemeshow test = 8.41; p = 0.394) (Figure 28).

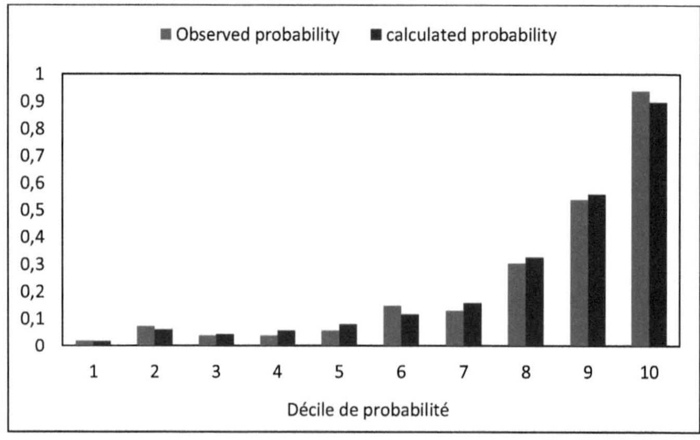

Fig. 28. Calibration of the neural model.

3.3.4.2. Logistic regression analysis

The univariate analysis showed that 12 variables were significantly associated with the occurrence of MI at the 20% threshold (age, sex, diabetes, hypertension, dyslipidaemia, personal coronary history, smoking, duration of symptoms, heart rate, ST-segment elevation, ST-segment sub-elevation and Q wave of necrosis), the threshold defined to retain these variables in the multi-variate step (table 16).

Table 16. Factors associated with MI. Univariate analysis by logistic regression.

Variables	Units	β	p
Age	years	0,0181	0,093
Gender	female = 0, male = 1	0,8266	0,002
Diabetes	no = 0, yes = 1	0,8435	0,002
HTA	no = 0, yes = 1	0,8765	0,001
Dyslipidemia	no = 0, yes = 1	0,9942	0,001
Personal history of coronary heart disease	no = 0, yes = 1	0,7807	0,061
Family history of coronary heart disease	no = 0, yes = 1	-0,2223	0,552
Former smokers	no = 0, yes = 1	0,7737	0,042
Current smokers	no = 0, yes = 1	1,1463	$< 10^{-3}$
Symptoms < 6 hours	no = 0, yes = 1	0,9555	0,002
Symptoms between 6 and 12 hours	no = 0, yes = 1	0,7306	0,031
NOT	mmHg	0,0043	0,489
PAD	mmHg	-0,0027	0,787

Heart rate	bpm	0,0423	$< 10^{-3}$
ST elevation	no = 0, yes = 1	1,4685	$< 10^{-3}$
ST sub-shift	no = 0, yes = 1	0,6873	0,035
Q wave	no = 0, yes = 1	2,5920	$< 10^{-3}$

The multivariate step of binary logistic regression identified eight predictors of MI (table 21): patient age (adjusted odds ratio [OR_a= 1.04; p = 0.009), being male (OR_a = 2.89; p = 0.004), having hypertension (OR_a = 3.18; p = 0.002), dyslipidaemia (OR_a = 2.69; p = 0.021), heart rate (OR_a = 1,06 ; p < 10^{-3}); and ECG disturbances, namely ST-segment elevation (OR_a = 8.25; p < 10^{-3}), ST segment sub-shift (OR_a = 4.65; p = 0.002) and the presence of a Q wave of necrosis (OR_a = 19,04 ; p < 10^{-3}).

The probability of having the IDM = 1/[1+exp (-y)]; or $y = -12.7219 + \Sigma\beta_i x_i$

Where the coefficients β_i represent the effect of the variable x_i adjusted for the effects of all the other variables included in the model. The variables x_i and β_i are listed in Table 17.

Table 17. Factors predictive of MI. Multivariate analysis by logistic regression.

	Variables	Units	β	OR$_a$	p
x_1	Age	years	0,0433	1,04	0,009
x_2	Gender	female = 0, male = 1	1,0616	2,89	0,004
x_3	HTA	no = 0, yes = 1	1,1576	3,18	0,002
x_4	Dyslipidemia	no = 0, yes = 1	0,9912	2,69	0,021

x_5	Heart rate	bpm	0,0611	1,06	$< 10^{-3}$
x_6	ST elevation	no = 0, yes = 1	2,1110	8,25	$< 10^{-3}$
x_7	ST sub-shift	no = 0, yes = 1	1,5365	4,65	0,002
x_8	Q wave	no = 0, yes = 1	2,9465	19,04	$< 10^{-3}$

Analysis of the Hosmer-Lemeshow test gives a Chi² value of 8.36 (p = 0.399), indicating good calibration (Fig. 29).

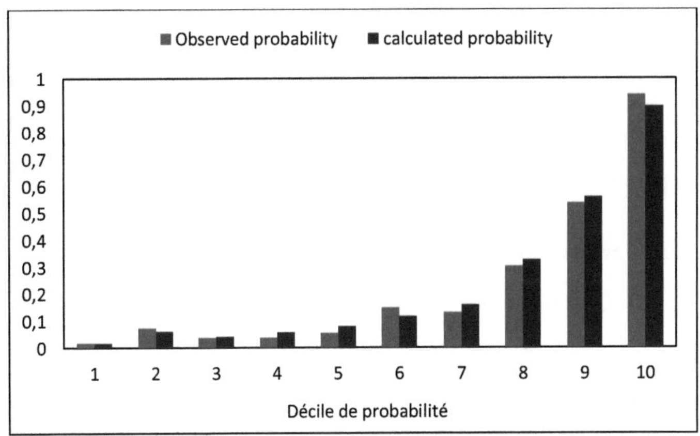

Fig. 29. Calibration of the logistic model.

A diagnostic score for MI was established by taking into account the eight variables mentioned above, according to their imputability (table 18).

Table 18. Diagnostic score for MI.

Variables	Points	Calculating the score
Age (in years)	1	Age in years
Gender (female = 0, male = 1)	25	+ 25 if male
HTA (no = 0, yes = 1)	30	+ 30 if high blood pressure
Dyslipidaemia (no = 0, yes = 1)	25	+ 25 if dyslipidemia
Heart rate (bpm)	1	+ Heart rate in bpm
ST elevation (no = 0, yes = 1)	50	+ 50 if ST elevation
ST sub-shift (no = 0, yes = 1)	35	+ 35 if ST sub-shift
Q wave (no = 0, yes = 1)	70	+ 70 if Q wave
		= Diagnostic score

The threshold was set at 235 in order to obtain the best sensitivity/specificity ratio. Thus, patients with a score of 235 or above are diagnosed with MI.

3.3.5. Comparative analysis of the performance of predictive models

3.3.5.1. Analysis of confusion matrices

The correct classification rate for the neural model was 94.4%. It was 95.2% for the data from the training sample and 92.6% for the data from the test group (table 19).

Table 19. Confusion matrix of the neural model.

		Total sample Predicted values			Learning sample Predicted values			Test sample Predicted values		
		IDM =0	IDM =1	Total	IDM =0	IDM =1	Total	IDM =0	IDM =1	Total
Observed values	IDM =0	414	8	422	294	3	297	120	5	125
	IDM =1	22	96	118	15	66	81	7	30	37
	TBM	94,4 %			95,2 %			92,6 %		

As for the logistic model, the rate of correct classification was 88.5% for all observations. It was 88.4% for the training group data and 88.9% for the test sample (table 20).

Table 20. Confusion matrix for the logistic model.

		Total sample Predicted values			Learning sample Predicted values			Test sample Predicted values		
		IDM =0	IDM =1	Total	IDM =0	IDM =1	Total	IDM =0	IDM =1	Total
Observed values	IDM =0	402	20	422	284	13	297	118	7	125
	IDM =1	42	76	118	31	50	81	11	26	37
	TBM	88,5 %			88,4 %			88,9 %		

3.3.5.2. Diagnostic performance analysis

The sensitivity and specificity of the neural model test group were 81.1% and 96% respectively. The PPV and NPV were 85.7% and 94.5% respectively (table 21).

Table 21. Diagnostic performance of the neural model.

	Total sample		Learning sample		Test sample	
	%	[95% CI]	%	[95% CI]	%	[95% CI]
Sensitivity	81,4	[65,9 - 99,3]	81,5	[71,3 - 89,2]	81,1	[64,5 - 92,0]
Specific	98,1	[96,8 - 99,4]	98,9	[96,9 - 99,9]	96	[92,6 - 99,4]
VPP	92,3	[87,2 - 97,4]	95,6	[87,8 - 99,1]	85,7	[69,7 - 95,2]
VPN	94,9	[92,9 - 96,9]	95,1	[92,7 - 97,5]	94,5	[90,5 - 98,4]

For the observations in the test sample, the logistic model had a sensitivity of 70.3%, a specificity of 94.4%, a PPV of 78.8% and an NPV of 91.5% (table 22).

Table 22. Diagnostic performance of the logistic model.

	Total sample		Learning sample		Test sample	
	%	[95% CI]	%	[95% CI]	%	[95% CI]
Sensitivity	64,4	[55,8 - 73,0]	61,7	[51,1 - 72,3]	70,3	[53,0 - 84,1]
Specific	98,1	[96,8 - 99,4]	95,6	[93,3 - 97,9]	94,4	[90,4 - 98,4]
VPP	79,2	[71,1 - 87,3]	79,3	[69,3 - 89,3]	78,8	[61,1 - 91,0]
VPN	9,5	[87,8 - 93,2]	90,1	[86,8 - 93,4]	91,5	[86,6 - 96,3]

3.3.5.3. Analysis of ROC curves

A comparison of the two models **in** terms of predictability shows the performance of the neural technique compared with logistic regression. Indeed, using all the observations, the area under the ROC curve of the neural model (AUC = 97.8%; 95% confidence interval [95% CI] = [96.2% - 98.9%]) was significantly greater than that of the logistic model (AUC = 91.1%; 95% CI = [88.3% - 93.3%]) (p< 10^{-3}) (Fig. 30).

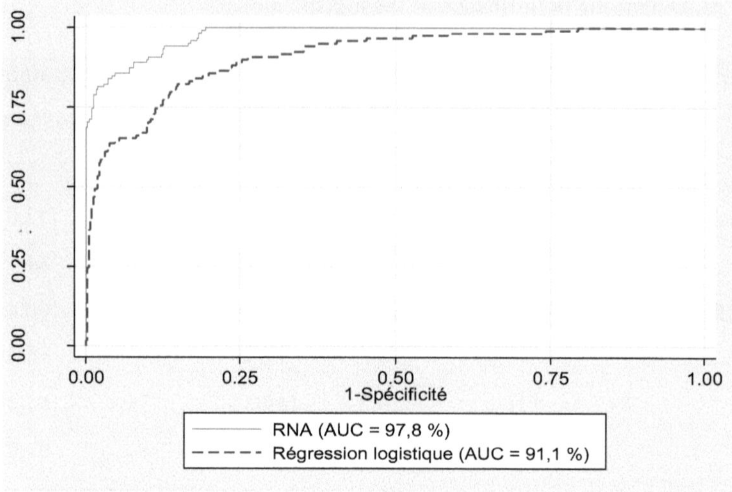

Fig. 30. ROC curves of the neural and logistic models for all observations.

The ROC analysis also showed the superiority of the neural approach over logistic regression, for both training and test data. In fact, for the training data, the AUC of the neural model was 98.2% (95% CI = [96.3% - 99.3%]) and that of the logistic model was 90.8% (95% CI = [87.4% - 93.5%]) (p < ') (Fig. 31). 10^{-3}) (Fig. 31). For the test data, the AUCs were 97.2% (95% CI = [95% - 99.3%]) and 91.2% (95% CI = [85.8% - 96.6%]) respectively (p = 0.0126) (Fig. 32).

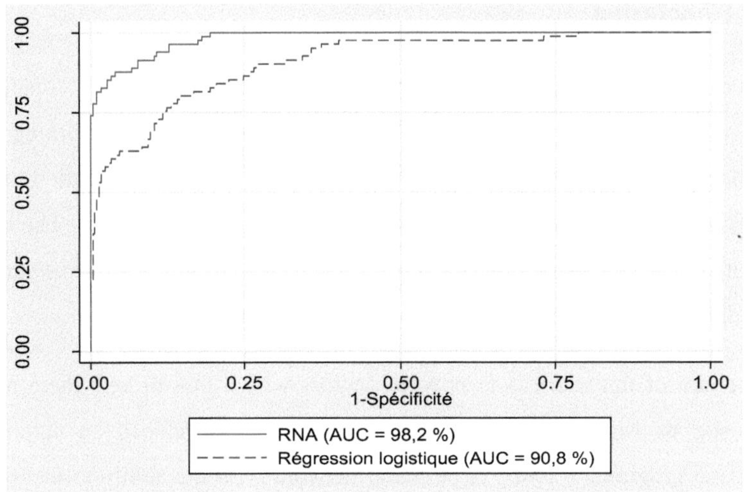

Fig. 31. ROC curves for the neural and logistic models of the training group.

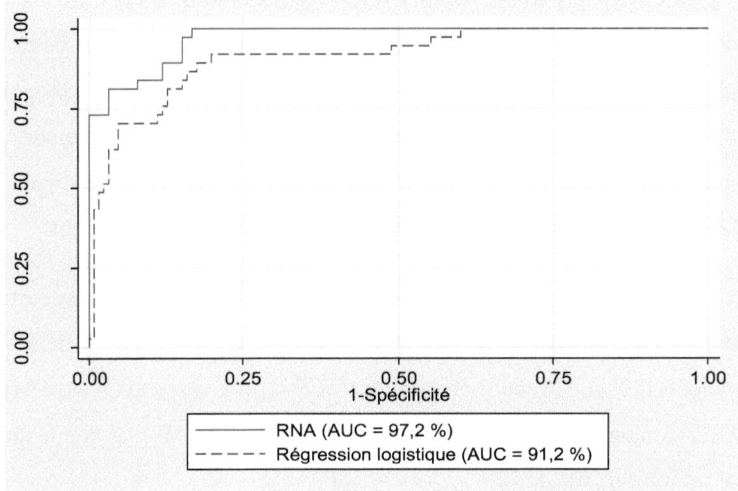

Fig. 32: ROC curves for the neural and logistic models of the test group.

4. Conclusion

Thanks to advances in IT tools, medical care and, more broadly, the biomedical field, research into intelligent medical systems and artificial learning has developed considerably, focusing on common challenges. The contributions made by this research have led to substantial improvements in patient care. The work presented in this thesis manuscript is part of this context, where we have studied an artificial learning algorithm in the context of predicting MI.

The aim of this work is to provide doctors with a tool to help them make diagnostic decisions. With this in mind, we have developed an automatic diagnostic programme based on a neural network with the ability to identify a patient with MDI. This discrimination is made by reference to a comparison value obtained by applying the algorithm in question. Experimental application of this algorithm has confirmed the validity and reliability of the technique.

Our predictive study was performed on 540 patients admitted to the cardiology emergency department of the EHU of Oran during the period from January to December 2015. The diagnosis of MI was retained in 118 patients, a proportion of 21.8%. A male predominance was noted with a sex ratio of 1.9. Cardiovascular risk factors were dominated by hypertension (41.5%), followed by dyslipidaemia (32.2%) and diabetes (30.5%). Smoking was reported in 22% of patients.

The mean time to emergency was 26.33 ± 21.3 hours, with extremes of 1 to 320 hours. ST elevation was observed in 71 patients (60.2%) and ST depression in 26 patients (22%). Seventy-one patients (60.2%) progressed to Q-wave MI and 47 (39.8%) to non-Q-wave MI. The topographical form of MI was dominated by anterior infarction (50%).

Sensitivity analysis using ANR identified nine variables predictive of MI, namely patient age, personal history of hypertension, dyslipidaemia and coronary heart disease, smoking status, heart rate, ST-segment elevation, ST-segment undershoot and the presence of a Q wave of necrosis on the electrocardiographic tracing. On the other hand, the multivariate stage of the logistic regression identified eight variables predictive of MI, namely the patient's age ($OR_a = 1.04$), being male ($OR_a = 2.89$), having high blood pressure ($OR_a = 3.18$), dyslipidaemia ($OR_a = 2.69$), heart rate ($OR_a = 1.06$); and ECG disturbances, namely ST-segment elevation ($OR_a = 8.25$), ST-segment elevation ($OR_a = 4.65$) and the presence of a Q wave of necrosis ($OR_a = 19,04$).

The results of the predictive analysis obtained prove that neural networks can be used to predict MDI in the emergency department with a sensitivity of 81.1%, a specificity of 96% and an area under the ROC curve of 97.2%. As for the diagnostic performance of logistic regression, sensitivity was 70.3%, specificity 94.4% and the area under the ROC curve 91.2%.

Thus, the neural network of the present study can be incorporated into computer programs and can detect the presence of pathology by means of input variables.

Compared with the logistic model, the neural approach seems to perform better in predicting MDI. Logistic regression remains a choice when the aim of model development is to examine the causal relationship between variables. However, ANNs may be better at prediction.

5. Bibliography

1.   WHO. Cardiovascular diseases. Fact sheet [Online]. January 2015 [Cited on. Available: http://www.who.int/mediacentre/factsheets/fs317/fr/index.html.

2.   INSP. Mortalité générale. TAHINA project. National Institute of Public Health. Algiers. 2005.

3   Charpentier S, Savary D, Lapostolle F, Chouihed T, Bonnefoy E, Manzo-Silberman S, et al. European Society of Cardiology recommendations for the management of patients with non-ST-segment elevation acute coronary syndrome. Annales françaises de médecine d'urgence. 2014;4:56-64.

4.   Body R, Cook G, Burrows G, Carley S, Lewis PS, Jarvis J, et al. Can emergency physicians 'rule in'and 'rule out'acute myocardial infarction with clinical judgement? Emergency Medicine Journal. 2014:emermed-2014-203832.

5   Lee TH, Rouan GW, Weisberg MC, Brand DA, Acampora D, Stasiulewicz C, et al. Clinical characteristics and natural history of patients with acute myocardial infarction sent home from the emergency room. Am J Cardiol. 1987;60:219-24.

6   Emerson PA, Russell NJ, Wyatt J, Crichton N, Pantin CF, Morgan AD, et al. An audit of doctor's management of patients with chest pain in the accident and emergency department. Q J Med. 1989;70:213-20.

7   Puleo PR, Meyer D, Wathen C, Tawa CB, Wheeler S, Hamburg RJ, et al. Use of a rapid assay of subforms of creatine kinase-MB to diagnose or rule out acute myocardial infarction. N Engl J Med. 1994;331:561-6. DOI: 10.1056/NEJM199409013310901.

8.   Roberts R, Kleiman NS. Earlier diagnosis and treatment of acute myocardial infarction necessitates the need for a 'new diagnostic mind-set'. Circulation. 1994;89:872-81.

9   Luepker RV. Delay in acute myocardial infarction: why don't they come to the hospital more quickly and what can we do to reduce delay? Am Heart J. 2005;150:368-70. DOI: 10.1016/j.ahj.2005.05.012.

10   McGinn AP, Rosamond WD, Goff DC, Jr, Taylor HA, Miles JS, Chambless L. Trends in prehospital delay time and use of emergency medical services for acute myocardial infarction: experience in 4 US communities from 1987-2000. Am Heart J. 2005;150:392-400. DOI: 10.1016/j.ahj.2005.03.064.

11   Azzaz S, Charbonnel C, Ajlani B, Cherif G, Convers R, Blicq E, et al, editors. Evolution of interventional management and reperfusion times in the acute phase of ST-segment elevation myocardial infarction. Annals of cardiology and angeiology; 2015: Elsevier.

12.   Le Breton H. Prise en charge de l'infarctus du myocarde: les délais. La Presse Médicale. 2011;40:600-5.

13   Atoui H. Conception de systèmes intelligents pour la télémédecine citoyenne: Villeurbanne, INSA; 2006.

14   Danchin N, Coste P, Ferrières J, Steg P-G, Cottin Y, Blanchard D, et al. Comparison of thrombolysis followed by broad use of percutaneous coronary intervention with primary percutaneous coronary intervention for ST-segment-elevation acute myocardial infarction. Circulation. 2008;118:268-76.

15   Wijns W, Kolh P, Danchin N, Di Mario C, Falk V, Folliguet T, et al. Guidelines on myocardial revascularization. European heart journal. 2010;31:2501-55.

16   Antman EM, Cohen M, Bernink PJ, McCabe CH, Horacek T, Papuchis G, et al. The TIMI risk score for unstable angina/non-ST elevation MI: A method for prognostication and therapeutic decision making. JAMA. 2000;284:835-42.

17   Ohman EM, Granger CB, Harrington RA, Lee KL. Risk stratification and therapeutic decision making in acute coronary syndromes. JAMA. 2000;284:876-8.

18   Xue J, Aufderheide T, Scott Wright R, Klein J, Farrell R, Rowlandson I, et al. Added value of new acute coronary syndrome computer algorithm for interpretation of prehospital electrocardiograms. J Electrocardiol. 2004;37 Suppl:233-9.

19   Harrison RF, Kennedy RL. Artificial neural network models for prediction of acute coronary syndromes using clinical data from the time of presentation. Ann Emerg Med. 2005;46:431-9. DOI: 10.1016/j.annemergmed.2004.09.012.

20   Green M, Björk J, Hansen J, Ekelund U, Edenbrandt L, Ohlsson M, editors. Detection of acute coronary syndromes in chest pain patients using neural network ensembles. Second International Conference on Computational Intelligence in Medicine and Healthcare; 2005.

21   Kennedy RL, Harrison RF. Identification of patients with evolving coronary syndromes by using statistical models with data from the time of presentation. Heart. 2006;92:183-9. DOI: 10.1136/hrt.2004.055293.

22   Ambalavanan N, Carlo WA. Comparison of the prediction of extremely low birth weight neonatal mortality by regression analysis and by neural networks. Early Hum Dev. 2001;65:123-37.

23   Engle RL, Jr, Flehinger BJ. Why expert systems for medical diagnosis are not being generally used: a valedictory opinion. Bull N Y Acad Med. 1987;63:193-8.

24   Kennedy RL, Harrison RF, Marshall SJ. Do we need computer-based decision support for the diagnosis of acute chest pain: discussion paper. J R Soc Med. 1993;86:31-4.

25   Drew PJ, Monson JR. Artificial neural networks. Surgery. 2000;127:3-11. DOI: 10.1067/msy.2000.102173.

26.   Baxt WG. Application of artificial neural networks to clinical medicine. Lancet. 1995;346:1135-8.

27.   Thygesen K, Alpert JS, Jaffe AS, Simoons ML, Chaitman BR, White HD, et al. Third universal definition of myocardial infarction. J Am Coll Cardiol. 2012;60:1581-98. DOI: 10.1016/j.jacc.2012.08.001.

28   Thygesen K, Alpert JS, White HD, Joint ESCAAHAWHFTFftRoMI. Universal definition of myocardial infarction. J Am Coll Cardiol. 2007;50:2173-95. DOI: 10.1016/j.jacc.2007.09.011.

29   Baxt WG, Skora J. Prospective validation of artificial neural network trained to identify acute myocardial infarction. Lancet. 1996;347:12-5.

30   Eggers KM, Oldgren J, Nordenskjöld A, Lindahl B. Diagnostic value of serial measurement of cardiac markers in patients with chest pain: limited value of adding myoglobin to troponin I for exclusion of myocardial infarction. American heart journal. 2004;148:574-81.

31.   Hajian-Tilaki K. Sample size estimation in diagnostic test studies of biomedical informatics. Journal of biomedical informatics. 2014;48:193-204.

32   Bhatt DL, Peterson ED, Harrington RA, Ou F-S, Cannon CP, Gibson CM, et al. Prior polyvascular disease: risk factor for adverse ischaemic outcomes in acute coronary syndromes. European heart journal. 2009;30:1195-202.

33   Diakite ANF. Etude épidemio clinique et thérapeutique des douleurs thoraciques non traumatiques aux urgences: Université de Bamako; 2011.

34.   Moreno L. Evaluation of the management of chest pain suspected of acute coronary syndrome in a chest pain unit emergency department: Toulouse III University; 2015.

35   Rumelhart DE, Hinton GE, Williams RJ. Learning representation by back-propagation errors. Nature. 1986;323:533-6.

36   Hunter A, Kennedy L, Henry J, Ferguson I. Application of neural networks and sensitivity analysis to improved prediction of trauma survival. Comput Methods Programs Biomed. 2000;62:11-9.

37   Hosmer D, Lemeshow S. Applied logistic regression. New York: Wiley; 1989.

38   Hanley JA, McNeil BJ. The meaning and use of the area under a receiver operating characteristic (ROC) curve. Radiology. 1982;143:29-36. DOI: 10.1148/radiology.143.1.7063747.

39   DeLong ER, DeLong DM, Clarke-Pearson DL. Comparing the areas under two or more correlated receiver operating characteristic curves: a nonparametric approach. Biometrics. 1988;44:837-45.

CONTENTS

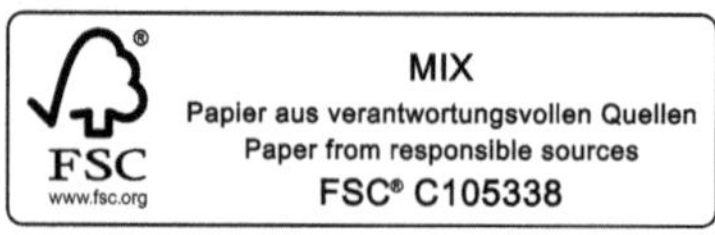

Printed by Books on Demand GmbH, Norderstedt / Germany